How to Improve Your Health and Fitness

333 Great Health and Fitness Tips for Busy Moms

By Judith Brown

Published by BizMove
www.bizmove.com

Table of Contents

1. Healthy Eating

Take a positive approach to making healthy changes in your diet and life-style. Instead of mourning what you're giving up, concentrate on all the benefits you're getting from your improved diet.

You can improve your chances for a long and healthy life by cutting down on the fat, salt, caffeine, and sugar in your diet. The average American eats 4 times more fat, 40 times more salt and caffeine, and 100 times more sugar than the body normally needs.

Eating a nutritious breakfast every morning and avoiding snacks between meals are 2 of the easiest ways to improve your eating habits. A balanced diet is a varied diet. It's best to eat many kinds of foods in order to ensure that your body gets all the proteins, carbohydrates, fats, vitamins, and minerals it needs. Vitamin and mineral supplements aren't necessary for most people. A well-balanced diet should provide you with all the vitamins and minerals required for good health.

Smoking destroys your body's supply of Vitamin C. Drink a glass of orange juice in the morning instead of lighting up a cigarette.

Eating between meals upsets the proper functioning of your metabolism. If you must snack, try raisins, nuts, apples, or crunchy vegetables instead of sugary foods.

Foods are most valuable to the body the closer they are to their natural state. Vegetables grown in your own backyard are superior to commercial frozen, canned, or dehydrated products. You can also home can, freeze, and dry your garden's surplus without any of the preservatives or additives found in many commercial products.

High-fiber vegetables, fruits, and whole grains are natural intestinal cleansers and also help to keep down the levels of cholesterol in the blood by binding up cholesterol and fats. Studies also show that a daily dose of bran in your breakfast cereal reduces the risk of bowel cancer.

Drink plenty of water daily. Water cleanses your system and promotes healthy-looking skin.

Sugar plays a role in the development of tooth decay, obesity, diabetes, and cardiovascular disease. If you do nothing else to improve your diet, at least cut down on your intake of sugar.

Cookies, cakes, and candies made with sugar provide only "empty calories" -that is, they have little nutritional value.

Add natural sugar to your diet by replacing baked goods and fattening desserts with fresh fruits.

When you need a pick-me-up, try drinking a glass of fruit juice or fresh, cold water instead of a sweetened soft drink Sugar is sugar, no matter what form it takes.

Don't be misled by "sugarless" products that contain corn syrup, honey, molasses, maltose, glucose, dextrose, and invert sugar. These are just other names for sugar. If you must avoid sugar for medical reasons, read labels carefully and be aware of the many names that sugar goes under.

Under normal circumstances your body needs no more than a teaspoon of salt a day. Too much salt in the diet can lead to high blood pressure, overweight, and heart and circulatory problems.

You can cut down on salt painlessly by leaving it out of your cooking, by removing the salt shaker from the table, and by using salt substitutes if you really miss the taste.

Substitute herbs, spices, and pepper in place of salt when seasoning foods.

Use lemon and lime juices to flavor vegetables in place of salt.

Reduce the salt content of instant broth by using twice as much water as the package directions indicate.

Many commercial canned foods contain high levels of salt. Canned soups are often especially high in salt. Read labels carefully.

A high-fat diet can be dangerous to your health. When cooking, consider using polyunsaturated fats such as corn, soybean, and sunflower oil instead of saturated fats such as lard, butter, chicken fat, coconut oil, or hydrogenated vegetable oils.

Low-fat skim milk contains considerably less fat than whole milk The same is true of skim milk cheeses, low-fat cottage cheese, and yogurt.

When buying meats, look for the leanest cuts. Trim off any visible fat before cooking, and whenever possible choose broiling over any other preparation method; broiling can reduce the fat content of meat by up to one-half.

Although broiling is the best cooking method for meat if you're trying to avoid fat) you can also substantially reduce the fat and calorie content of meat by boiling or pot-roasting it and skimming off the fat.

You can improve your whole family's diet by beginning to replace some meat dishes with fish and poultry. You'll be eating less fat and fewer calories.

Legumes) especially peas and beans) are an excellent source of protein and should be included in your weekly menus.

Experiment with meatless meals to cut down on your fat intake. Meatless spaghetti sauce) chili) and vegetable soup can taste just as delicious as the meaty versions.

Whole-grain bread) pasta) potatoes) and rice and other grains are good energy foods and sources of protein.

Avoid eating too many preserved meats such as ham) hot dogs) and corned beef. Processed meats contain chemical additives.

Don't toss away the darker outer leaves of your lettuce head. They're higher in nutrients than the leaves found closer to the core.

Scrub vegetables with a vegetable brush to remove any surface dirt before cooking. Don't remove the skins) because you'll also be throwing out most of the vitamins and minerals.

Cook your vegetables briefly by steaming them. Overcooked vegetables lose their Vitamin C and mineral content.

Be sure your child's diet contains lots of milk and milk products) as well as enriched breads and green) leafy vegetables. These foods are high in calcium} which is essential in building strong bones and healthy teeth.

Accustom your children's taste buds to non-sugared foods by preparing their breakfasts with sugar-free cereals. Sweeten with raw honey) sliced bananas} chopped apples} or raisins.

In place of candy} potato chips} and pretzels} give your youngsters healthy snacks like sun-flower seeds) raw almonds or cashews) roasted soy nuts} or fresh or dried fruits.

Fry your foods in a nonstick pan which requires no additional oil for frying.

Cut out as much sugar as possible from your diet in the summer. Mosquitoes are attracted to people who eat a lot of sugar.

If you're often out in the sun} stay away from caffeine drinks such as coffee) tea} or cola. Caffeine makes your skin more sensitive.

Eat smaller meals more often in summer. Your body will have to work less to digest the foods, and you'll feel cooler.

Use more salt in your foods during the summer months, especially if you perspire a lot.

Heavy perspiration depletes the salt content of your body.

If you're susceptible to colds, fortify your diet with extra Vitamin C by drinking lots of fruit juice or rose-hip tea.

To keep your bones from getting brittle as you get older, be sure that your diet is rich in calcium from milk products and Vitamins A, C, and D which are present in citrus and vegetable juices.

A tablespoon of brewer's yeast added to a glass of fruit or vegetable juice or milk acts as a natural laxative.

Substitute honey for sugar as a sweetener. It serves as a natural laxative.

To calm an upset stomach, drink a glass of buttermilk or skim milk mixed with a tablespoon of cider vinegar.

When you're pregnant, follow these tips:

* To control weight gain during pregnancy, cut down on sweets but not on whole-grain bread and potatoes which you need for energy.

* To reduce feelings of nausea during pregnancy, try eating only cold foods.

* If you can't tolerate any other foods in the morning, at least eat bread or dry toast with milk

* To ensure that your diet contains a good supply of Vitamins A and D, eat liver or an oily fish such as herring, sardines, or mackerel once a week.

* To prevent constipation, eat fiber-rich foods such as whole-grain breads and lots of fresh fruits and vegetables.

* To control nausea, take small sips of cola or bites

of bland food, such as custard, gelatin, or mashed potatoes, throughout the day.

* Nibbling on nuts, cheese, or other high-protein foods every 2 to 3 hours can * help relieve feelings of nausea in early pregnancy. Substitute frequent nutritious snacks for three heavy meals a day.

* Eating a cracker with a glass of milk before bedtime helps reduce heartburn and ensures a sound sleep.

2. Healthy Lunchtime Ideas

Freeze a carton of yogurt overnight and take it to work with you. The yogurt will be thawed but still cold by lunchtime the next day; it's a delicious, low-calorie lunch.

You can fix lunches for the entire week on Sunday night. Hard-boil a dozen eggs and fry 2 chickens. Then wrap each piece of chicken securely in plastic wrap and divide these prepared foods

into lunch bags, with a different piece of fruit and cheese for each day of the week. Store the bags in the refrigerator and take one out each morning on your way to work.

You can make and freeze sandwiches up to 2 weeks ahead of time, provided you use no jelly, mayonnaise, eggs, lettuce, or tomato in the filling.

Butter the bread, add the sandwich filling, and wrap the sandwiches tightly in plastic wrap before storing in the freezer. A sandwich removed from the freezer in the morning will be ready to eat by lunchtime.

If your work place offers nowhere to keep your lunch refrigerated during hot weather, freeze sandwiches containing mayonnaise or salad dressing the night before, even though mayonnaise separates when it's frozen. The sandwiches will thaw by lunchtime without spoiling from the heat.

Plan well-balanced box lunches. Include a protein-rich food, a crisp fruit or vegetable, a beverage or soup, and a treat.

Make extra servings of chili and stews to use in your lunch box. Pour them hot into vacuum containers for eating the next day, or freeze in serving-size portions for later in the week.

Freeze cartons of prepared shrimp or crab cocktail. They'll thaw out but still be cold by the time you're ready to eat lunch.

Good fillings for pita bread are grated cheese, cottage cheese mixed with tomatoes, onions, and cucumbers, a spread made from chickpeas, or pate. Add plain yogurt and shredded lettuce just before eating.

To prevent soggy sandwiches, moisture-proof your sandwich bread by spreading on a thin layer of margarine or butter before adding the filling.

For more food value-and to give you more energy-make lunch-time sandwiches from whole-grain breads and buns instead of white bread.

You can cut down on calories at lunch (or at any other time) by eating hamburgers and sandwiches open-faced, with only one slice of bread or bun.

A 40-ounce plastic freezer container provides the perfect lunch box for carrying salad fixings to the office. Add a low-calorie dressing of lemon juice and herbs just before eating your salad. If the salad is dressed ahead of time it will go limp.

You can avoid that mid-afternoon slump that usually follows close on the heels of a heavy lunch by sticking to salads or light foods at lunch time.

Try to use part of your lunch hour to visit a museum, do some shopping, or take a lunchtime exercise class-the break will refresh you more than a long, sedentary lunch.

Fill plastic sandwich bags with an assortment of fresh vegetable sticks for a light vegetarian lunch, or for snacks to nibble if you're trying to avoid sugar-laden between-meal snacks.

A packet of powdered skim milk provides a quick, vitamin-packed, liquid lunch food. It's also a real source of protein, calcium, and Vitamin B2.

Keep a mouthwash concentrate in your purse or desk to mask the scent of any onions or garlic eaten at lunch. Better yet, keep toothbrush and toothpaste at work and make a habit of brushing your teeth after lunch.

For an eat-on-the-run lunch) mix 1 fresh egg yolk into a glass of orange juice. Add a teaspoon of honey to sweeten.

Even if you're in a hurry) don't gulp down your lunch. You'll only get indigestion later. Eat slowly) chewing your food well.

Instead of taking a coffee and doughnut break) take an exercise break instead. Treat yourself to a handful of raw seeds or nuts afterward.

Several ice cubes sealed with a twist tie in a plastic bag is an easy ice bag for keeping your lunch cold.

3. **Ideas for Weight Watchers**

Gaining or losing weight is basically a matter of addition or subtraction. Each pound on your body is worth 3500 calories. In order to lose 1 pound) you must cut back by 3500 calories. In order to gain 1 pound you must increase your food intake by 3500 calories.

Despite extravagant claims by certain advertisers and certain health clubs) vibrating machines) body massages) saunas) and steam baths won't really reduce your weight. You'll lose a lot of body fluid because of perspiration) but the fluid will return as soon as you drink water.

Don't expect to lose weight through exercise alone. Sensible dieting will help you lose weight) and exercise will help you maintain a firm) healthy body.

If you're in the habit of eating while you're busy doing something else) such as watching TV or reading) make an effort to stop doing so. Making just a single change in your snacking habits can help you shed unwanted pounds.

Instead of spending extra money on diet foods or low-calorie items, eat what you normally do but eat less of it.

A glass of water can fill you up enough to distract you from hunger pangs and help you resist between-meal snacks.

If you're having trouble losing weight) avoid having in the house 'instant' foods that can be eaten without extensive preparation. The thought of having to spend time preparing foods may deter you from eating them.

Cutting down on alcohol can significantly reduce the amount of calories you take in. For some people it's possible to lose weight simply by eliminating alcohol from the diet altogether.

If you're on a diet) it may help to turn after-meal cleanup over to somebody else. That way you won't be tempted to munch on leftovers as you're putting them away.

Keep a record of everything you eat, and it'll be easier to reinforce your goals for weight loss.

The record will also be a reminder of how often you are cheating on your diet.

If you eat your meals with someone whose

company you enjoy, you'll probably talk more and eat less.

When you're tempted to have a second helping of some food, tell yourself you can have it in 5 minutes. During the 5 minutes, keep busy doing something else. You'll probably forget about wanting the extra food.

Use smaller plates for your diet-size meals.

Smaller portions look more satisfying on a proportionately smaller plate, and you won't feel that you're on starvation rations. The same strategy applies to wine glasses and dessert dishes.

When you're on a diet, foods that take longer to eat can be more satisfying than easy-to-eat foods. For example, corn on the cob seems like more than the same amount of cut corn, and lobster in the shell will keep you busy longer than a boneless steak.

When making stews and other dishes containing grease or fats, prepare them ahead and then store them in the refrigerator. The fat will rise to the surface, where you can easily lift it off before reheating and serving the dish.

Substitute yogurt for whipped cream or artificial

dessert toppings.

Substitute club soda or mineral water for an evening cocktail. Eat fresh vegetables from a relish tray instead of fattening hors d'oeuvres.

Dieters can snack, too, if their diet allows for it. There are many snacks that fall under 100 calories. Try 5 ounces of ginger ale over a peeled and sectioned orange. Or add a sprits of orange and lemon to tomato juice, then blend with ice cubes. Or prepare raw vegetables along with 1/3 cup of plain yogurt splashed with herbs for dipping.

To cut down on calories, season your vegetables with lemon juice and herbs instead of butter.

Dips made from packaged mixes pack a weighty wallop of calories, but it isn't the mix that makes them fattening-it's what they're mixed with. Most packaged mixes add only 50 calories, but the directions call for a base of sour cream (485 calories per cup) or cream cheese (850 calories in an 8-ounce package). You can cut calories dramatically by substituting plain, unsweetened yogurt -only 130 calories-for sour cream or the low calorie, low-fat "imitation" cream cheese-only 416 calories-for the real thing.

If you check the nutrition information printed on competing packaged products and choose one with the lowest calorie count, you can save calories the same way a cost-conscious shopper saves money.

The lower the fat content in dairy products, the fewer calories they contain. For example, cottage cheese that's labeled 99 percent fat-free has only 160 to 180 calories a cup, while regular creamed cottage cheese has 240 to 260 calories.

The word "imitation" on low-calorie, low-sugar, or low-fat products doesn't necessarily mean that the product is made up of chemicals, only that the lower sugar or fat content keeps the product from conforming to standard recipes.

Often the imitations are more nutritious than the real thing. For example, some low-sugar jams and preserves contain more fruit and less sugar, and some imitation low-fat cheeses have a higher protein content.

If you drink 1 sugar-sweetened cola per day, you could lose nearly 15 pounds in 1 year by substituting a diet drink-or by eliminating the cola altogether.

Lean Canadian bacon is a better choice for dieters than regular bacon, which is more than half fat even after it's been broiled or fried and well-drained. Canadian bacon contains only 45 calories an ounce compared with 200 for regular bacon.

A cup of plain herbal tea (no cream or sugar) makes a no-calorie, no-caffeine, low-cost beverage.

For a low-calorie lunch, roll your sandwich filling into lettuce leaves instead of using 2 slices of bread.

A low-calorie substitute for sour cream: Mix cottage cheese in the blender until smooth and flavor it with herbs.

If you're on a special diet and are taking a plane trip, call the airline 24 hours in advance to ask them if they can accommodate your dietary needs instead of serving you their regular menu.

To avoid gorging yourself at holiday parties, drink a glass of skim milk or eat a piece of fruit before you go. This will take the edge off your appetite and help you resist the urge to devour everything in sight once you get to the party.

If you don't want to be tempted by leftovers from your own party, offer guests the option of taking a doggie bag home.

4. **Exercise and Fitness**

Vigorous exercise brings both mental and physical benefits. Not only does it send more blood to the heart and improve the heart's pumping activity, but it makes you feel relaxed and less likely to crave cigarettes, alcohol, and junk foods.

Walking, biking, swimming, or jogging are among the best forms of aerobic exercise. Whichever you choose, it should be something you enjoy. Otherwise, you won't get the mental benefits -and you probably won't stick with it very long anyway.

If you take in more calories than you burn up, you'll soon be overweight. In order to lose weight,

you must combine sound nutrition with vigorous exercise-at least 20 minutes of aerobic exercise, 3 times a week. Exercising strenuously 1 day a week can do more harm than good and won't make up for not exercising on a steady basis during the rest of the week.

Design an exercise program for yourself that helps to tone each part of the body: arms, chest, waistline, legs, and abdomen. Always do warm-up and cool-down exercises as part of your daily regimen.

If running, swimming, bicycling, dancing or other forms of exercise don't appeal to you, you can include exercise in your life in more routine activities: Get off the bus or train a few blocks ahead of your stop and walk briskly the rest of the way. Don't get out the car for short trips; walk instead. Walk up and down stairs instead of taking the elevator. Get up a little earlier and take a 15-minute walk before breakfast. Take a walk during your lunch break each day.

Take the pinch test for fatness: If you can pinch more than an inch of fat in the fold of skin just above your hipbone, you could use an exercise program.

Carry a sweater or sweatshirt to wear after exercising, but don't put it on immediately after you finish. Wait until you've cooled down a bit, or you may actually interfere with the body's normal efforts to eliminate excess heat.

Exercise helps ward off heart problems. People who lead sedentary lives are twice as susceptible to heart attack as those who exercise regularly.

Exercise is good for practically everyone, regardless of age. But if you've been leading an inactive life, don't plunge into a rigorous exercise program without checking with a doctor. You need to start slowly and build up stamina by means of a graduated exercise program. This is especially true for older people.

Don't exercise for an hour after eating a full meal. Otherwise you can exercise any time that suits your schedule.

Try to exercise at the same time every day so that exercising becomes a habit. If exercise has become a regular part of your routine, you'll be less likely to skip sessions on off days when you just don't feel like making the effort.

Avoid the "weekend athlete" syndrome. If you sit around all week and then exercise energetically on weekends you're likely to strain your heart.

Also avoid the "vacation athlete" pattern. If you're inactive for 50 weeks of the year and try to make up for it on vacation you could wind up in the hospital. At any rate, you'll be exhausted because your body is not accustomed to exercise, and any benefits you do gain will be dissipated within a short time of returning to your sedentary life. It's a good idea to drink an 8-ounce glass of water before you exercise.

If you're a runner, you should also drink on the run-a glass of water for every 5 miles you cover.

Always warm up and cool down your body before and after exercising to lessen the chance of injury or muscle strain. Sit-ups and leg-stretches should be included in any series of warm-up stretches. You can cool down nicely by finishing off your exercise period with some walking.

Try this deep-breathing routine to warm up for exercising: Standing straight with your arms at your sides, rise up on your toes while making small circles with your arms as you raise them over your head. Inhale deeply while doing this movement. Then, exhale slowly as you lower your arms to your sides and lower your heels.

Here's another good ,"arm-up exercise: Stand with your feet together and your hands on your hips, then jump from side to side for a minute; this will get your circulation going and loosen your muscles.

While exercising, wear comfortable clothing that doesn't restrict your body movements. Wear clothing made of a natural fiber like cotton, which breathes and lets perspiration evaporate.

To condition your body for skiing, practice the following exercise: Hold on to the edge of a chair and extend your right leg in front of you at least 1 foot off the floor. Lower your body to a squatting position without letting your leg touch the floor. Come up again to your original standing position and repeat this sequence with your left leg extended. Alternate 5 times with each leg.

Regular exercise in the form of physical work or formal exercise not only keeps you fit but helps you sleep well at night. If you have trouble sleeping, try getting more exercise during the day so that you're healthily tired by bedtime.

When doing any aerobic exercise, use the "talk test" to determine whether you're working at the proper rate. If you can't talk normally while exercising, it means you're working too hard and too fast.

Walking briskly is excellent for your heart, lungs, and general muscle tone. Walking at a good clip burns off 360 calories an hour.

Whenever you drop something during the day, do either a deep knee bend or a toe-touch while retrieving it.

Buy a heavyweight rope at the hardware store and skip rope while you watch the nightly news or your favorite television program. To benefit your heart and circulation, set up non- stop for 5 minutes. Or try running in place for 5 minutes.

For floor exercises, soften the hard surface with a mat or a large towel.

To tone your entire body and increase your circulation, stand up straight with your elbows bent at shoulder level. Pump your arms as you gently jump your legs up to your chest. Alternate and lift each leg at least 5 times.

Bicycling is a good overall body conditioner and benefits both your respiration and your leg muscles.

Swimming strengthens your leg, arm, back, and abdominal muscles.

Don't jog immediately after eating a meal or in very hot or cold weather. Running tracks and grass are the safest surfaces for your feet. If you can, avoid running on concrete.

Exercising in any extremes of humidity and temperature can cause strain. Remember to take it easy and rest frequently. On very hot and humid days or on very cold days, it may be advisable to skip exercising.

Stop exercising if you feel chest pain or shortness of breath. If either condition continues longer than 5 minutes, get medical attention.

Don't continue to exercise if you suffer a strain or a sprain. Give your body a chance to recuperate by taking a rest from physical activity for a few days.

Sneakers don't provide your feet with enough support for jogging. You could injure yourself by running in sneakers instead of in comfortable running shoes that have firm soles, a good arch support, and flexibility. The correct gear is worth the investment.

Women should wear specially designed sports bras for added support and protection when jogging.

When jogging, wear cotton clothes that allow perspiration to evaporate. Rubberized or plastic garments will make you sweat more initially, but can eventually produce chills.

In cold weather, insulate your feet by wearing 2 pairs of socks. Wear a nylon or rayon pair with a heavy cotton or wool pair on top.

The following exercises will help make you feel good all over:

* Take a tip from cats, who are among the most supple, athletic creatures alive, and stretch when you get out of bed in the morning. Stretching loosens the muscles and lengthens the spine to relax you and improve your posture.

* Sit on the edge of the bed and drop your upper torso between your legs, then slowly arch your back and raise your arms toward the ceiling; hold for 5 seconds.

* Lie on the edge of the bed, then raise your left leg and swing it over your right leg, trying to touch the toes of your left foot to the floor. Move to the opposite side of the bed and do the same exercise, this time swinging the right leg over the left leg.

* After your shower or bath, rub your body vigorously with a bath towel. This not only increases the circulation, but also improves your skin tone by sloughing off dead skin cells.

" Stand on 1 foot without any extra support while you put on your shoes and socks or stockings. This strengthens your leg muscles and improves your balance.

* To stretch tense back muscles, extend your leg at waist height onto the back of a chair or a window sill. Reach for your ankle with both hands and stretch as far as possible while you bend your knee slightly. Hold for 5 seconds, then repeat with your other leg.

* To stretch and strengthen your back and legs, sit on the edge of the bed and pull the knee of your right leg up to your chest, clasping both arms around the back of the leg. Slowly extend your leg forward, keeping it as straight as possible, then slowly lower it back down to the floor. Repeat with your left leg, alternating leg stretches 6 times .

* Sit on the edge of the bed with your feet flat on the floor. Take a deep breath while you raise your shoulders up to your ears. Exhale slowly while you lower your shoulders and relax. Repeat 3 times.

* To improve overall balance and muscle tone, stand up straight and bring your right knee up to your chest, grasping your lower right leg with both hands. Pull your thighs as tight to your chest as you can, keeping your back straight. Hold this position for 10 seconds, and then repeat with your left leg.

* If you tend to sit all day at your job, stand every once in a while-to make your phone calls, perhaps. Changing position is good for your circulation and bone structure.

Facial exercises:

* To strengthen and tighten your neck muscles, break into a wide grin as you tense your neck muscles. Repeat 10 times.

* To firm up your cheek muscles, open your mouth wide as if you were about to scream. Hold this position for several seconds, then relax. Repeat several times.

* To strengthen the eye muscles and smooth the skin around the eyes, open your eyes as widely as possible and hold them open. Look to the right, then to the left, then up and down for several seconds each. Close your eyes to relax, then repeat the movements 5 times.

* To reduce laugh lines around your mouth, pucker up as if you're about to whistle and hold this position for a few seconds, then relax. Pucker up 10 times.

* To exercise your jaw muscles, put your lips into a

pucker and move them in a circular direction for 5 seconds.

* Smile often during the day. It's a great easy way to exercise your facial muscles. Also, it will make you- and the people around you-feel more cheerful.

* To prevent age lines around your mouth, fill your cheeks with air and press your fists against your cheeks without releasing any of the air. Count to 10, then blowout the air slowly. Repeat the sequence 10 times.

* To slim a double chin, stick out your chin and pull your lower teeth over your upper teeth. Turn your head as far as it will go to the right, then as far as it will go to the left.

* You can lift your facial muscles by holding your cheeks tightly with your hands, then moving your mouth from side to side as far as it will go.

* Exercise your facial muscles by opening your mouth and eyes as wide as you can, then holding this position for 10 seconds. Next, squeeze your face as tightly as you can for 5 seconds, then relax.

* Yawning is one of the best exercises of all for your facial muscles, and it also forces you to get

more fresh air into your lungs.

Exercises to slim your waist:

* Standing straight with your feet wide apart, stretch your arms at shoulder level and twist your upper torso to the right and then to the left, going back and forth for a total of 20 counts. The twisting motion in this exercise helps to slim your waistline.

* You can trim a thick waist by practicing this simple exercise daily. Scatter matches on the floor and pick them up one by one without bending at the knees.

* Stand with your feet slightly apart and your arms straight out at shoulder level. Touch your right hand to your left toe, then touch your left hand to your right toe, alternating 10 times for each hand.

* Stand up straight with your feet slightly apart. Place your right hand on your hip and stretch your left hand over your head, bending your upper body over your right arm. Alternate with your left hand on your hip and bending to the right; repeat 10 times on each side .

* To help reduce waistline bulge, do this exercise regularly: Stand with your hands on your hips and

bend as far as possible to the right, then as far as possible to the left, bend to each side at least 10 times.

* With your left hand on your hip and your right hand straight up in the air, stand with your weight on your left leg and raise your right leg to waist - high level. Bend over and try to touch your toes with your right hand. Return to your original position and repeat with your opposite arm and leg, raising and lowering each leg 10 times.

* When doing toe-touching exercises, you'll be come winded quickly unless you breathe properly. Do it this way: Inhale, then exhale as you bend forward. As you straighten up, breathe in again.

Exercises to flatten your stomach:

* Exercises to firm your stomach create a natural girdle by strengthening the muscles that crisscross your abdomen. When you strengthen your stomach muscles, you may find it also helps to ease problems with a bad back. If your stomach muscles have been too slack, the back muscles have been carrying the extra load.

* Sit with your hands behind you on the floor and

your legs bent at the knees in front of you. Extend your legs, pointing your toes toward the ceiling, then return to your original position. Repeat this movement 6 times.

* Work on keeping your stomach in shape: While you're watching TV, tighten the muscles of your diaphragm, relax, and repeat several times.

* Sit on the floor with your feet spread apart in front of you, then lift your legs several inches off the floor and cross them in a scissors kicking motion several times. This exercise does wonders for flabby stomach muscles.

* Lie on a slant board, with your head down and your feet elevated 12 to 15 inches. Draw in your stomach while you count to 10, then relax.

* Lie on your back with knees bent, then come up to a sitting position. Lie back down and repeat the sit-ups at least 10 times. You can vary this by doing the whole exercise with arms folded across your chest.

* Here's a quick stomach toner that you can do sitting down. Start with your feet flat on the floor, then lift your knees to waist level and extend your

legs straight forward. Lower both feet slowly back to the floor. Repeat 10 times.

Exercises to slim the hips and thighs:

* To trim your inner thighs, hold on to something solid (like the kitchen counter) and swing your left leg out to the side as high as it will go. Repeat this movement several times, alternating right and left legs.

* Lie on your back, lift your hips up off the floor and support your hips with your arms. Move your legs in a pedaling motion as if riding a bicycle, and continue for 2 to 3 minutes.

* From a standing position, bend your knees to a 45° angle, keeping your feet flat on the floor, then return so a standing position. Repeat 20 times.

* Sit up straight in a chair with your hands holding onto the sides. Lift your left leg waist high and hold it straight in front of you for 5 seconds. Lower your leg, then repeat with the right leg. Alternate right and left legs at least 5 times each.

* Lie on your left side with your legs straight and your arms stretched out above your head on the floor. Lift your right leg as high as possible, and

lower it slowly back down to the floor, to a count of 5. Roll over and lie on your right side and repeat the sequence with your left leg. Alternate sides so that you raise and lower each leg at least 5 times.

* Holding on to the back of a kitchen chair and standing straight, bend your knees slightly, push your right leg behind you until you feel the muscles in your leg pulling, tightening the muscles of your buttocks as you push the leg back. Repeat with the other leg.

* This exercise is so easy you can do it either standing or sitting just about anywhere. Tighten your buttock muscles and hold for 3 seconds, then relax. Repeat 10 times.

* To trim excess fat from flabby hips, get on your hands and knees and extend your left leg sideways as high as it will go. Then repeat the same motion with your right leg. Alternate legs and repeat 10 times with each leg.

* To firm your buttocks, lie on your stomach with your legs together and your arms close to your sides. As you inhale, raise both your legs as high as possible and hold for 5 seconds. Lower them slowly while exhaling. (Don't do this one if you've had

lower back problems.)

* Lie on your stomach with your hands placed comfortably under your chin. Raise each leg as high as possible, moving it in a small circle. Then roll over onto your back and repeat the sequence with each leg. Exercises to strengthen the back and improve the posture:

* Good posture when you're both standing and sitting can help avoid back strain and fatigue. If your chair is uncomfortable, prop a cushion behind your lower back to support your spine.

* To increase flexibility in your lower back, stand with your feet slightly apart and your arms raised overhead. Bend forward from the hips and swing your arms downward between your legs. Repeat 5 times.

* If your job requires you to stand all day, shoes with heels over 2 inches high will throw your pelvis out of line and cause backache by the end of the day. Stick to lower heels and be comfortable.

* To relieve back tension and strengthen back muscles, get down on all fours, then slowly round your back like a cat. Hold for a few seconds and

then relax your back completely.

* When carrying luggage or packages, try to carry two smaller parcels rather than one heavy one. This helps balance the weight and prevent back strain.

Exercises to strengthen chest, shoulders, and upper arms:

* You can firm your breasts by practicing this exercise daily. Place your hands at eye level against a doorjamb and draw your hands together as hard as you can, lowering your hands down to waist level as you push.

* To strengthen chest and arm muscles, clasp your hands together close to your chest and push your palms together as hard as you can. Hold for 5 seconds.

* Lie face down on the floor with your palms facing down at shoulder level. Pushing off against your hands, raise your body off the floor, keeping your elbows straight. Lower yourself back to the floor and repeat as many times as you can to strength- en arm, chest, and shoulder muscles.

* Tone your chest and arm muscles by vigorously polishing something such as your car, a glass table,

all the mirrors in the house.

* To firm the bust, sit with your feet flat on the floor, with your arms folded across your chest. Raise your arms to chest height and press your arms as far to the right and then to the left as possible, repeating 25 times in each direction.

* Your arms and shoulders will get a good workout if you sit in a chair with your hands grasping the sides. Push yourself up and out of the chair with your arms, then lower your body back down into the chair. Repeat 3 times.

* Extending your arms with clenched fists over your head, make tiny circles in the air, keeping your arms rigid. Widen the circle gradually to hip level. Stretch your arms out in front of you and relax.

* Lying face down on the floor with arms tucked under your chest, push your upper torso up off the floor. It's important to keep your hips on the floor. Lower yourself and repeat 6 times.

* Scrubbing pots and pans using a vigorous circular motion helps to firm your upper arms.

* Digging and hoeing in the garden or raking leaves are good activities to strengthen and firm your

upper arms.

* To firm flabby upper arms, raise your elbows to shoulder level, then swing your arms back and forth. a Stand with your arms extended straight out to the sides, palms open toward the ceiling. Make a tight fist, hold for 3 seconds, then relax.

* Strengthen arm muscles by extending your arm over your head, bending your elbow, then stretching down toward the middle of your back as if to pull up a zipper.

Exercises to strengthen the legs, ankles, and feet:

* To tone and firm your calves, place your toes on the edge of a stair step and push down against your heel, pushing up and down rapidly 10 times; then repeat with your opposite foot. Do this on a bottom stair so you won't tumble too far if you lose your balance for a moment.

* To exercise your leg muscles after sitting for a long time, cross your right foot over the left, pressing the right heel against your left instep. Cross your legs in the opposite direction and repeat.

* To exercise your leg muscles and increase

circulation to the legs, climb the stairs 2 at a time.

* To refresh your legs after prolonged sitting, hold on to a countertop or the back of a chair and quickly bounce from heel to toe 25 times. ☐ To strengthen and slim your ankles, sit in a chair and move your feet in an arc while keeping your heels on the floor. Do 10 arcs, then relax.

* Exercise your feet and strengthen the arch of your foot by kneeling with your toes bent forward. Then sit back on your heels for 5 seconds.

* To revive tired feet at the end of the day, stand on your toes and roll onto the outer edges of your feet, back onto your heels, then onto the inner edges, ending up on tiptoe. Repeat 10 times.

* To strengthen foot muscles, walk alternately on your toes, on your heels, on the outsides of your feet, and on the insides of your feet.

* To increase the amount of circulation to your feet while you're seated, circle your foot at the ankle, making 5 complete circles in each direction.

* To give your feet a quick pick-me-up after sitting for a while, remove your shoes and place the weight of your leg on the heels and raise your toes. Move

your feet in a circular motion from the ankle for a count of 15, then change the direction of the circle.

* To strengthen tired ankles and feet, stand with your knees slightly bent and your head and back rounded forward. Roll onto the outside arches of your feet and hold this position for 5 seconds before returning to your original position. Repeat 5 times.

If you're planning to join a health club, note the following tips:

* Keep in mind that a health club membership is a long-term undertaking. You won't get your money's worth unless you go regularly-2 or 3 times a week.

* Don't join a health club that's more than about 20 minutes' journey from your home or workplace. Too much traveling will waste time (and gas) and make it easier to make excuses to yourself for skipping sessions when it all seems too much like hard work. If the health club is nearby, it won't be such an effort to get there.

* If there isn't a health club in your vicinity, check out the local YWCA or YMCA. The equipment may be less varied or sophisticated, but you'll still

get a good workout. Also, some high schools make their running tracks or swimming pools available to nonstudents outside of school hours.

* If you know yourself to be a reluctant exerciser, join a group or go to classes rather than rely on your own motivation. The structure will help you stay on task.

* When you're checking out a health club, visit it during the hours when you would expect to make use of its facilities yourself. If you plan to work out on the way home from work, for instance, visit the club at that time. If all you see is wall-to-wall people, look elsewhere. Overcrowding means you are likely to waste time waiting to use the equipment.

* Don't sign a health club contract without reading the small print. Will you get your money back if you decide to quit? And are there any hidden costs you should know about?

* Health clubs sometimes offer 1fz-price or 2-for-1 specials at certain times of the year. You'll obviously save money if you take out membership during one of these special-offer promotions.

Here's some useful advice about exercising during pregnancy:

* While you're pregnant, remember to walk tall and watch your posture. You'll feel less tired if you move around with the weight of your body distributed evenly.

* When you're sitting down, support your back and, whenever possible, put your feet up.

* Elevating your legs as often as possible during the day helps guard against varicose veins. So does wearing support stockings.

* To ease leg cramps during pregnancy, wear low heeled shoes and go barefoot whenever possible. Here are some good general exercises for a pregnant woman:

* Lie down, pressing your back against the floor. Pull your knees up to your chest and tighten the muscles of your buttocks, then relax. Repeat 5 times.

* Lying on your back with your hands above your head, press your back against the floor and raise your pelvis. Relax and repeat 5 times .

* Lying on your back with your knees bent toward your stomach roll your knees to the right and then to the left, rolling to each side 5 times.

Exercises for those over 50:

* To improve overall flexibility, sit in a chair and place a scarf firmly under your foot and pull up on your toes several times. Repeat with the other foot.

* To keep your waist flexible, sit in a chair and swivel your upper torso to the right and then to the left, keeping your hands at your side.

* To reduce swelling in your ankles, cross your right leg over your left leg. Press your toes up, down, in, and out, then move them in a circular motion. Uncross your legs and repeat with your left leg crossed over the right.

* To strengthen your back and spine, sit upright in a chair. Then draw your back up against the chair, throwing your chest out and keeping your head up. Hold for a few seconds, then relax and repeat.

* To flex your neck muscles, let your head fall forward, then lift it up and lean it first to the right and then to the left side.

5. Coping with Tension and Stress

While you can't eliminate stress, you can learn to manage too much stress before it creates serious physical or emotional problems. Exercise is a good tension reliever. Deep breathing and meditative relaxation can also help you cope.

Any exercise you do for 30 minutes or more will calm your nerves and reduce stress.

Take an exercise break the next time you feel tension and stress mounting, whether at work or at home. Shoulder rolls, head rolls, shaking the wrists, arm circles, and taking several deep breaths are some of the easiest and most effective stress relievers.

If you're tense because you've been sitting too long, stand with feet apart and raise your arms up over your head. Bend from the waist and try to touch your palms first to your right foot and then to the left foot. Raise your arms back over your head and relax.

To relax tense shoulder and neck muscles, lie on your back and arch your chest and shoulders until the top of your head is resting on the floor. Hold for 5 seconds and then relax.

To reduce tension in your neck, arms, and shoulders after prolonged sitting clasp your hands behind your chair and raise them as high as possible. Lower and repeat 5 times.

Another good stress relief exercise: Hunch your shoulders up toward your ears, keeping your muscles tense for a few seconds. Relax and repeat several times.

To help reduce shoulder tension while driving, grip the steering wheel tightly and raise your elbows as high as possible to the side; raise and lower them 10 times, then relax.

To relieve back tension while driving try this exercise while waiting at a stoplight. Grip the steering wheel and round your back, then slowly arch your back as far as possible, holding this position for 5 seconds before you relax. Keep repeating this movement until the light changes.

To relax a stiff neck, stand with knees bent slightly. Lean your right ear toward your right shoulder, then roll your head back toward your left shoulder, coming full circle and dropping your chin on your chest. Repeat 5 times.

To reduce tension in the head, neck, and shoulder region, stand or sit with hands resting in your lap. Drop your chin onto your chest as you raise your elbows as high as possible. Lower your elbows and lift your head to the starting position. Repeat 5 times.

To loosen stiff neck muscles, clasp your hands behind your neck and push as hard as you can. Repeat this contraction 5 times.

Another way of relieving neck tension: Let your head fall forward, then roll it clockwise and counterclockwise several times.

To relax tense shoulders, sit up straight and rest your fingertips on your shoulders. Then pull your elbows back as far as possible. Repeat several times.

The yoga slant. can help relax tense muscles and straighten your spine. Elevate a 12-inch wide by 6-foot long board by propping the lower end 12 to 15 inches off the floor. Recline with your feet in the elevated position for 15 minutes daily.

For an overall relaxer after exercising, lie on your

back with arms relaxed at your sides. Working from your toes up to the top of your head, concentrate on making each part of your body go limp.

To relax tired leg muscles, sit in a chair and extend your right leg out in front of you, flexing your foot inward. Bounce your leg up and down 15 times, then repeat with the left leg. This also helps trim ankles and calves.

To relax your entire body, lie on your stomach with your legs bent, your feet resting on your bottom. Grasp your ankles with your hands, then raise your head and chest up as you pull your legs toward the top of your head. Hold this position for 10 seconds, then relax.

Suffering from a pounding tension headache? Relax in a very warm bath. Warm water draws blood away from the head and helps reduce the pressure that's causing your headache. If you wake up feeling tense and tired,

take a warm shower and rub some rose oil on your arms and neck. You'll feel the tenseness in your muscles melt away. You can get the rose oil from the drug store.

If you feel tired at mid-afternoon during the work day, slump forward in your chair and sit with your head between your knees for a minute or two.

Getting a good night's sleep does wonders for your mental attitude and sense of physical well-being. Make sure you get as much sleep as you need.

Engaging in some physical activity during the day will help you to sleep better at night.

Exercise acts as a natural tranquilizer. Do not, however, exercise to the point of exhaustion.

Before bedtime, avoid eating rich, spicy foods, or taking caffeine drinks such as coffee, cola, or tea. Drink a cup of warm milk instead.

Reading before bedtime will help make you drowsy enough to sleep. It's also a good idea to keep a book on your night table so you can read yourself to sleep again if you awaken in the middle of the night.

Don't smoke in bed. Not only could you fall asleep before extinguishing your cigarette, but smoke fumes in the air may prevent you from getting a restful sleep.

If you're bothered by street light coming in at the windows, buy blackout shades. You won't be disturbed by the dawn's early light the next morning, either.

Once you're in bed, tense and relax each of your muscles, working from your feet all the way up to your face. This will help to relax your body, and you'll drift off to sleep easily.

If you awaken in the middle of the night and feel restless, drink a cup of warm milk mixed with a spoonful of brandy or sherry.

Cold feet can keep you awake. Wear bed-socks or use a hot water bottle.

Place a board under your mattress for a firmer sleep foundation.

Some people find that soaking in a hot tub relieves tension. It's important to remember, however, that you must observe safety precautions when using a hot tub.

To eliminate any danger of electrical shock, have a local building inspector double-cheek the installation of your hot tub.

Use a tested, reliable thermostat in a hot tub. Defective thermostats can be seriously inaccurate.

To be on the safe side, never enter a hot tub alone. This is particularly important for those who have a health problem such as epilepsy, high blood pressure, or diabetes.

If the temperature in a hot tub rises 2 degrees above 104°F; heat stroke could set in. The maximum temperature for adults should be 100°F; for children under age 5 the maximum should be 98°F.

Don't enter a hot tub if you've been drinking alcohol, or if you have taken a tranquilizer. There have been cases of people who became so drowsy and relaxed that they slid under the surface of the water and drowned.

When you're pregnant, don't soak in a hot tub if the water temperature is over 100°F. You may damage your unborn child.

Don't stay too long in a hot tub. After 15 minutes your body may overheat and your blood pressure drop dangerously.

After sitting in a hot tub, don't shock your system by going directly into cold water such as that of a swimming pool.

6. **Health Care and First Aid**

If you need to find a family doctor, poll your friends, neighbors, and relatives for recommendations. A hospital nurse, intern, or resident who has actually observed or worked with a doctor should also be able to give you a fair assessment of that doctor's capabilities.

Although you may be impressed by a doctor who's on the staff of several hospitals, remember that such a physician may not always be as available as who isn't so heavily committed.

It is usually safe to assume that a doctor affiliated with a university teaching hospital is highly qualified. However, be sure that the time your doctor must spend in teaching and lecturing doesn't take away from the amount of time he or she can spend on general practice.

Don't be hesitant about asking your doctor for clarification or explanation of your health problem or the prescribed treatment. It's true that a doctor's time is valuable, but it's part of the doctor's job to help you to be an informed partner in your own health care. The better informed you are, the better able you'll be to follow the doctor's orders.

If a doctor consistently fails to answer questions to your satisfaction, or to spend as much time with you as you can reasonably expect your health care to require, look for another doctor.

Be sure to ask your doctor whether generic drugs, which are less expensive than brand-name drugs, can be used to fill your prescription. Also ask your doctor for booklets or other literature on the use and possible side effects of prescribed drugs.

If you're scheduled for surgery, find out if all the required lab tests can be done prior to your admittance. You can save hundreds of dollars by shortening a hospital stay by even 1 day.

Avoid going to a hospital emergency room for treatment unless it really is an emergency. You'll pay 2 or 3 times more than you'd be charged for a visit to your doctor's office.

Mornings and early afternoons are often the best times for scheduling a doctor's appointment.

At those times appointments are more likely to be running closer to schedule. In any case, call your doctor's office before leaving home for an appointment and ask if the doctor is running on schedule.

The receptionist may suggest you come a little later rather than wait at the doctor's office.

You can make your own cough syrup by mixing 1 teaspoon of honey with 1 teaspoon of lemon juice.

Unless your sore throat is severe, you can often treat it at home. Gargle every couple of hours with a glassful of warm water mixed with tea-spoon of table salt. Keep warm, drink plenty of fluids, and rest.

Many people are allergic to pollens, molds, and house dust. Air conditioning can lessen your contact with pollen. Keeping your kitchen, laundry and bathroom areas scrupulously clean helps prevent the spread of molds, Regular dusting and vacuuming will keep down the house dust too, particularly if your vacuum cleaner has a filter. Air cleaners can also help ease the discomfort of allergy sufferers.

If you take aspirin, avoid taking it before or after drinking orange juice. The combination can be damaging to the stomach.

Wearing rings while you, wash the dishes can lead

to skin irritation because detergent becomes trapped under your rings. Take your rings off before you start the cleanup.

If washing dishes makes your hands rough, wear protective rubber or vinyl gloves whenever you have to put your hands in water. When cleansing your hands, use vegetable or mineral oil instead of soap.

Keep your adhesive bandages in the refrigerator. The cold will make the backing easier to peel off.

After first putting a bandage in place, don't disturb it for the next 24 hours. After that time, you can change the dressing as often as needed.

If you are trying to pinpoint the cause of an eye condition, remember that allergies cause itching and tearing, but never pain or pus. Viruses cause pain and tearing, but not pus. Foreign bodies cause pain, sensitivity to light, and tearing, but there'll be no pus and the redness will be confined to one part of the eye.

You can treat heat rash by keeping the area dry and applying calamine lotion. Wear light, loose clothing that won't further irritate the skin.

Cold, not heat, will help relieve a toothache.

Repeated soaking in warm Epsom salts solutions (⅛ cup per quart of water) can bring a boil under control.

To avoid straining your back, always bend your knees when reaching down to pick up an object.

If your feet swell in the summer heat, bathe them in tepid water and rinse them with cool water. Splash with bracing cologne and dust on talc. Sprinkle talc inside your shoes, too.

Soak tired feet in warm water and Epsom salts. Then lie down with feet elevated for 10 or 15 minutes.

Pat the skin around a splinter with baby oil or olive oil; the splinter will slide out more easily.

If you feel movement on your skin, but can't see anything, you may have a mite infection.

Moisten a piece of sterile cotton with rubbing alcohol and press it to the skin for a minute or two.

Have a dermatologist examine the cotton in order to make a diagnosis. If you do have mites, call an exterminator. The presence of mites usually indicates that there are mice in the house.

If you have a special health problem, wear a tag identifying your health problem and listing your doctor's phone number and the names of any medications you are taking. Also carry an identification card in your wallet. In an emergency, even if you're unconscious, those caring for you will be better able to treat you promptly and correctly.

Bees are attracted to hair spray, bright colors, and perfume. If you are stung, remove the stinger and wash the spot. Then dissolve 1 teaspoon of meat tenderizer in 2 tablespoons of water and rub this mixture on and around the stung area. Another way to get relief from an insect bite is to pat the area with a cotton swab dampened with aromatic spirits of ammonia. If the swelling is severe or the victim suffers other symptoms, get medical attention immediately.

You can probably drive an ill person to the hospital faster than an ambulance could-since you won't have to wait for the ambulance to arrive.

Call an ambulance or rescue squad only in a life-threatening situation or when no other transportation is available.

Fast action is important if a harmful liquid or powder gets in the eye. Hold the eye open and flush it with water. Then get immediate professional attention.

Juice from a broken rhubarb stalk helps relieve the pain of an insect bite.

You can take the sting out of an insect bite by applying an ice-pack for a few minutes and then applying calamine lotion.

To stop a bleeding cut, press the wound hard with a clean compress. After the bleeding has stopped completely, wash the cut gently with a mild soap under running water.

You can minimize bruising if you apply cold compresses soon after an injury has occurred.

After 24 hours a bruise will tolerate warm applications, which will hasten healing.

To stop a nosebleed, sit with your head tilted back, breathe through your mouth, and pinch your nose.

To treat chemical burns, immediately wash the area for 5 minutes with running water. Then apply a clean dressing and seek medical attention.

To treat a burn in which the skin is blistered but unbroken, immerse the burn in cold water or wrap the area in cold, wet towels. Do not apply grease or butter to a burn.

Patting sunburned skin with a wet teabag or a cloth dampened with vinegar provides relief. Or tie 6 to 8 teabags together and add them to a tepid bath for all-over sunburn relief.

Another way to ease sunburn is to bathe in lukewarm water to which you've added bicarbonate of soda.

If you're bitten by an animal, wash the area with soap and water and have the injury checked by a doctor. If you can do so without risking further injury, capture the animal alive to have it checked for rabies.

If someone has suffered an electric shock, locate the source of power and shut it off before touching the victim. If you can't break electrical contact, pull the person away from the source of power by using a dry rope, a wooden pole, or a loop made from clothing or fabric.

To treat sunstroke, move the victim immediately to

a cool, shady spot. Give the victim a glass of water and place an ice pack on his or her head. If the victim's temperature is below normal, keep the person warm and call a doctor.

Most people don't realize that accidents are most likely to occur in their own homes. Accident-proof your home by identifying and correcting any possible hazards.

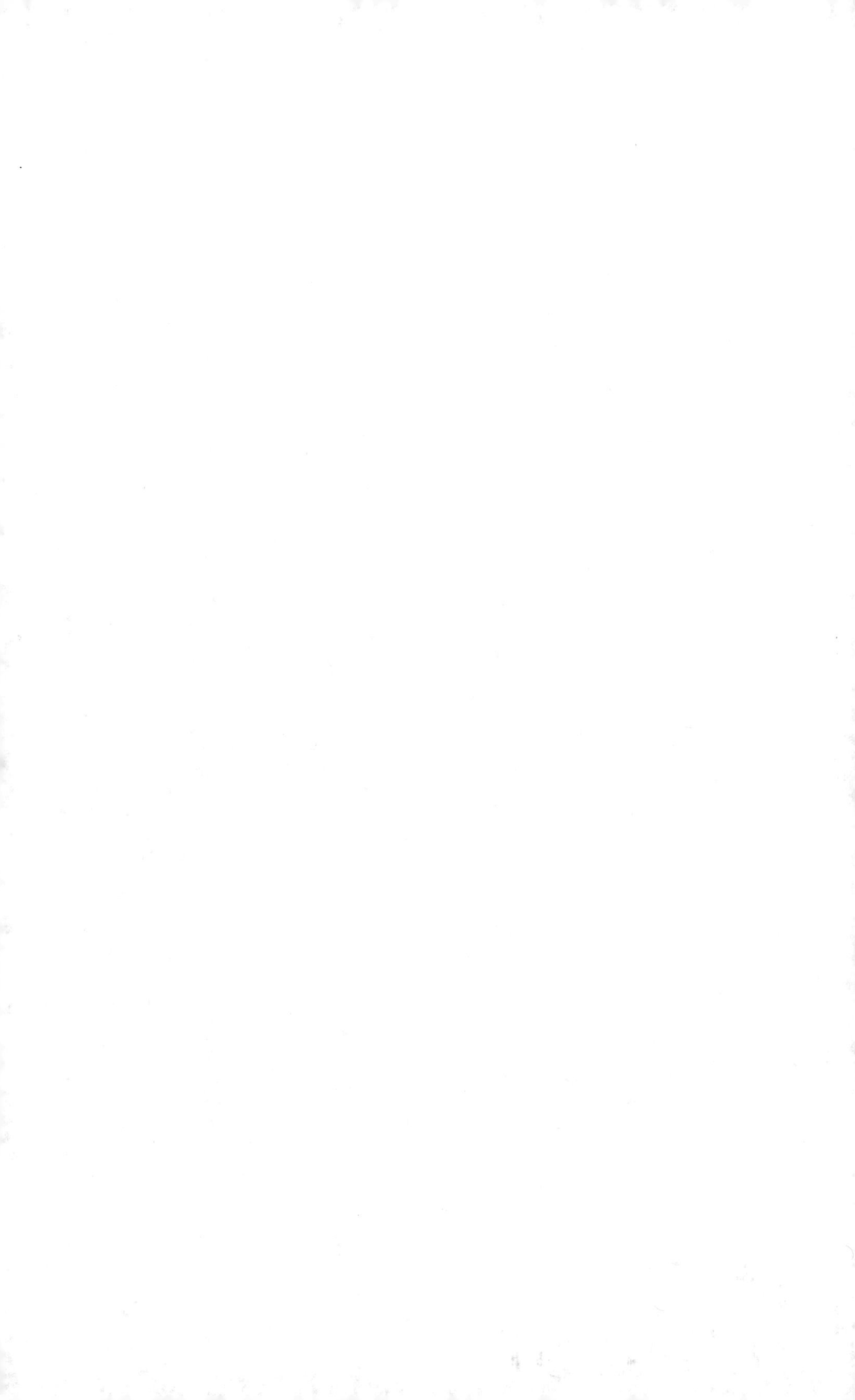

www.ingramcontent.com/pod-product-compliance
Lightning Source LLC
Chambersburg PA
CBHW070828240726
48654CB00007B/510